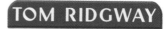

TOM RIDGWAY

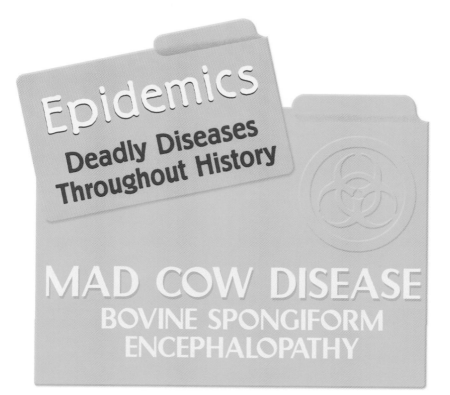

Epidemics
Deadly Diseases
Throughout History

MAD COW DISEASE
BOVINE SPONGIFORM
ENCEPHALOPATHY

The Rosen Publishing Group, Inc.
New York

To BHL, who ate it, too

Published in 2002 by The Rosen Publishing Group, Inc.
29 East 21st Street, New York, NY 10010

First Edition

Library of Congress Cataloging-in-Publication Data

Ridgway, Tom.
Mad cow disease: bovine spongiform encephalopathy/
by Tom Ridgway.— 1st ed.
p. cm. — (Epidemics)
Includes bibliographical references and index.
ISBN 0-8239-3487-X
1. Prion diseases—Juvenile literature. 2. Bovine spongiform encephalopathy—Juvenile literature. [1. Mad cow disease.
2. Prion diseases. 3. Diseases.] I. Title. II. Series.
RA644.P93 R535 2002
616.8—dc21

2001002150

Cover image: An electron micrograph of prion fibrils in the brain of a cow infected with BSE, or mad cow disease.

Manufactured in the United States of America

CONTENTS

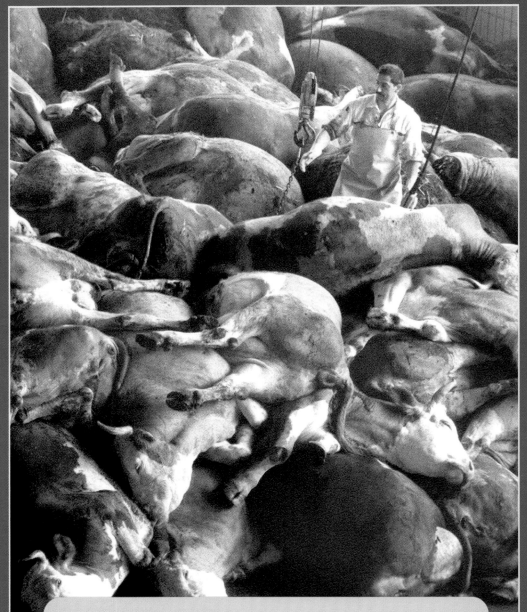

Bovine spongiform encephalopathy, more commonly known as mad cow disease, is a fatal condition that affects cows and humans.

INTRODUCTION

One day, in the south of the United Kingdom, Cow 133 started acting very strangely. She started shaking her head, acting more aggressive than usual, and having a lot of trouble walking—as though she didn't know where to put her feet. When she died, in February 1985, scientists did some tests and found something that they hadn't seen before. The cow, they said, had been killed by a "novel progressive spongiform encephalopathy."

Cow 133 was the first cow diagnosed with bovine spongiform encephalopathy, commonly referred to as BSE. The name isn't actually as hard to understand as it is to pronounce. Bovine means "relating to cattle" (from the Latin for

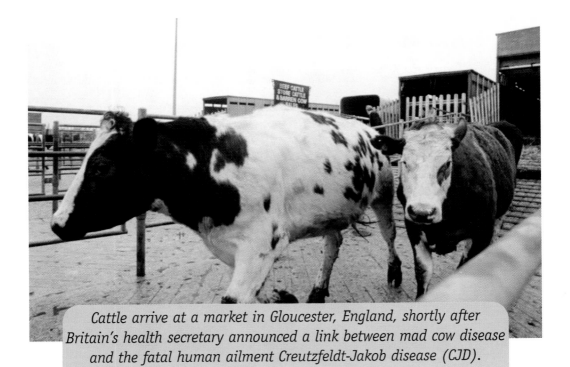

Cattle arrive at a market in Gloucester, England, shortly after Britain's health secretary announced a link between mad cow disease and the fatal human ailment Creutzfeldt-Jakob disease (CJD).

ox); spongiform means "being full of holes," like a sponge; encephalopathy means "a disease that affects the brain" (from the Greek words *enkephalos*, meaning "brain," and *pathos*, meaning "suffering" or "disease"). The name is pretty much self-explanatory: BSE is a disease that affects cattle by making their brains look like sponges. When this happens, the brain begins to develop tiny holes and stops working as it should. The more holes there are, the less the brain works—until the animal dies.

Of course, with a long name like bovine spongiform encephalopathy, it's no surprise that the media quickly came up with another one—mad cow disease.

If the disease had continued to affect only cattle, it might not have been too worrisome. After all, sheep have been victim to a similar disease for over 200 years without there being any grave consequences. But in 1995—ten years after the first case of BSE—Stephen Churchill, a nineteen-year-old Englishman, died of a rare brain disease. When someone dies from a strange or unknown disease, doctors perform what is called a postmortem (or autopsy), where they look inside the body to see how the person might have died. When a postmortem was performed on Stephen Churchill, the doctors realized that Stephen had died from a disease that no one had ever seen before. Though it looked a lot like another disease called Creutzfeldt-Jakob disease, or CJD, Stephen Churchill's disease was slightly different. The doctors had to find a new name, and they decided to call it new variant Creutzfeldt-Jakob disease, or nvCJD.

The doctors were worried because Stephen's brain looked more like the brain of a cow that had died of BSE than a brain of a human who had died of a typical case of CJD. It seemed as though the disease that had started killing cows ten years earlier had somehow been passed on to humans—a frightening scenario considering that the only way that Stephen could have caught his horrible disease was from eating beef infected with BSE. Even more frightening was that there were probably hundreds of thousands—if not millions—of British people who had also eaten beef that came from infected cows.

Since the scientists knew that the disease came from cows, and they knew what it did to people, one might assume that it would have been easy to find a cure. However, this was not the case. BSE and nvCJD aren't as simple as you may think. They're new diseases, and it takes scientists a long time to properly understand (and to understand how to treat) new diseases. And that's not all: The infectious agent—the thing that damages the brain—is a mystery. In fact, it's such a mystery that even twenty years after its discovery, some scientists can't quite seem to believe that it actually does exist.

Before we go any further, it's only fair to warn you: This is not a book for the squeamish. We're going to have to talk about experiments on animals, about how animals are killed so that we can eat them, and about what we do with the bits of animals that we don't eat. And there aren't going to be many neat and simple answers either, because not even the world's best scientists have got them.

HOLES IN THE BRAIN

When scientists first wrote about BSE in 1985, they called it a "novel progressive spongiform encephalopathy." Novel means that it was a new disease, progressive means that it gets worse as time passes, and as we've seen, a spongiform encephalopathy is a disease that kills by attacking the brain. BSE was the newest member of a known group of diseases called transmissible spongiform encephalopathies, or TSEs. (If you get confused about all of these acronyms, be sure to look at the glossary on page 57.) The different diseases in the group all have similar symptoms—those who are infected become antisocial, experience difficulty walking and balancing, and lose weight. The other common thing about TSEs is, whether infecting

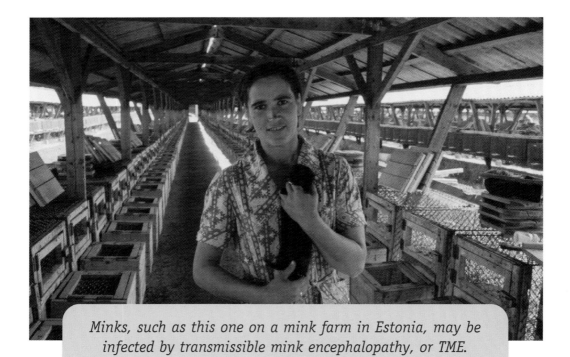

Minks, such as this one on a mink farm in Estonia, may be infected by transmissible mink encephalopathy, or TME.

a sheep or a human, once one is infected with a TSE, there's only one result: death.

Scientists know that TSEs infect humans and animals who live on farms or near humans. However, this doesn't mean that TSEs don't infect other animals. It's just that scientists and researchers haven't come into as much contact with these cases.

Other Well-Known TSE Cases

⊛ Transmissible mink encephalopathy, or TME, affects mink. Usually, this disease breaks out on mink farms where the animals are reared for their fur. (It may also affect wild mink, but there has not been any research conducted on wild mink.) The first reported case of TME was on a ranch in Wisconsin in 1947. The last outbreak was in 1985, when over 4,300 mink on a farm (again in Wisconsin) died. The disease has also been found in mink in Canada, Finland, Germany, and the former republics of the Soviet Union.

Chronic wasting disease, or CWD, was first spotted in 1967 in a herd of deer living at a research facility that bordered northern Colorado and southeastern Wyoming. The disease also infects elk, and since the first outbreak, it has affected wild deer and elk in the same part of the country.

Lastly, and most important, there's scrapie, which was first spotted in sheep in England and Scotland over 200 years ago. The first case in the United States was in 1947, and now the only two countries in the world that are said to be free of the disease are Australia and New Zealand. The disease makes sheep act like any other animal infected with a TSE, but it also makes sheep bite their legs and feet, smack their lips, and sometimes hop like rabbits. There is one sure sign that a sheep is infected, which is also how the disease got its name: Infected sheep start to scrape themselves against fixed objects, such as trees, gate posts, or

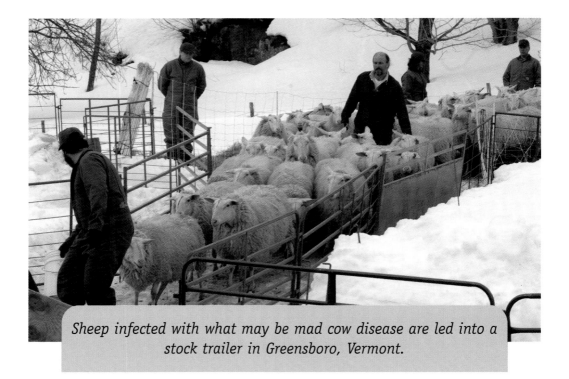

Sheep infected with what may be mad cow disease are led into a stock trailer in Greensboro, Vermont.

fences. Sometimes they rub themselves so much that they scrape off not only their wool but also their skin. The symptoms of the disease do not start to appear until two to five years after the sheep has been infected, but once a sheep starts showing symptoms, it will live for only another one to six months.

Human TSE

The first human TSE—Creutzfeldt-Jakob disease—was discovered in 1920 by Hans Gerhard Creutzfeldt, a German doctor. A year later, another German doctor, Alfons Jakob, came into contact with four more cases, and so the disease was named after both doctors. Every year, the disease affects about one person in every million, which means that there are about 250 cases in the United States each year. CJD is a disease that affects mainly older people; the average age of CJD victims is sixty-five years old.

Scientists have found that there are three different ways that CJD infects and kills people. The most common— affecting 85 percent of cases—is sporadic CJD, meaning that the disease attacks people randomly. Five to 15 percent of cases are hereditary CJD, meaning sufferers inherit a susceptibility from their parents. In fewer than one percent of cases, the

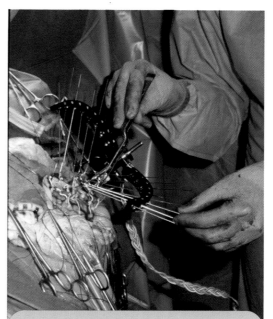

Surgical procedures (such as brain surgery) using improperly sterilized electrodes have helped spread CJD.

disease is caught: This is called acquired CJD. In the past, cases of acquired CJD have occurred following certain brain or eye operations. For example, patients became infected following surgical procedures where electrodes that were not properly sterilized were placed in their brains. Cases have also been found to result from contaminated growth hormone. During the late 1960s and early 1970s, growth hormone was taken from the pituitary gland (a small sac at the base of the brain that produces the hormone that controls growth). Growth hormone was often taken from the brains of dead people, processed, and then injected into people who had not grown properly. Sometimes, however, the hormone became infected with CJD and the patients who received the hormone eventually died from the disease. (The hormone is now created artificially, so there should be no more infections because of it.)

Kuru—the Human TSE

Apart from CJD, there are three other types of human TSEs. There's Gerstmann-Straussler-Scheinker (GSS) and fatal familial insomnia (FFI), both of which are exceptionally rare inherited diseases. Then there's kuru.

Kuru first appeared in the early 1900s among the Foré people, a tribe that lives in what is now Papua New Guinea. In the 1950s, the Foré numbered 8,000. Between 1957 and 1968, 1,100 Foré died from a mysterious disease that they called *kuru*, which means "to shiver" or "to tremble" in their

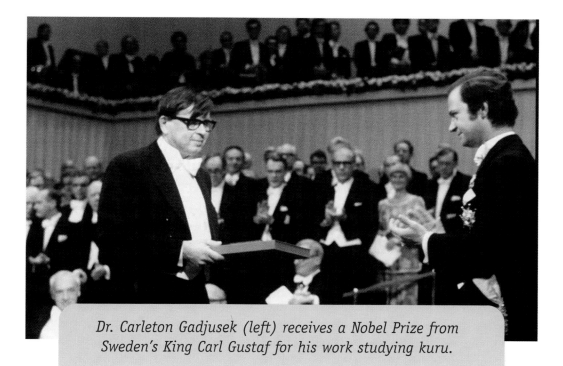

Dr. Carleton Gadjusek (left) receives a Nobel Prize from Sweden's King Carl Gustaf for his work studying kuru.

language. Eight times more women than men died of the disease, and scientists who went to investigate couldn't understand what was going on. At first, it was thought that the disease was hereditary, but then Dr. Carleton Gadjusek, an American doctor, performed some experiments that suggested otherwise. Dr. Gadjusek injected bits of the brains of people who had died of kuru into monkeys, and, eventually, the monkeys died in the same manner as the humans had. Having established that the disease was infectious (meaning that it could pass from person to person), Dr. Gadjusek knew that the

1985
Cow 133 dies of a strange brain disease after suffering from tremors, weight loss, and incoordination.

1987
Infected meat-and-bone meal (MBM) is identified as the source of BSE.

1986
Bovine spongiform encephalopathy (BSE) is identified as a disease by the British government.

1988
MBM is banned in the U.K. It is announced that all infected cattle will be slaughtered.

1990
British agriculture minister John Selwyn-Gummer claims that British beef is safe to eat, feeding his daughter a hamburger in front of journalists.

spread of kuru must have had something to do with the lifestyle of the Foré.

The Foré were cannibals; they ate people. When a Foré died, the Foré women would perform a ritual whereby they would remove the arms and the feet from the dead body, strip the arms and legs of the muscle, remove the brain, and cut open the chest in order to remove internal organs, such as the heart. The Foré men ate the muscles, and the Foré women and children ate the other parts—including the brain (it was thought to make them smarter). Dr. Gadjusek realized that this practice of eating people who had died of the disease was in fact passing the disease on.

1992
The British government sets up the National CJD Surveillance Unit to keep track of Creutzfeldt-Jakob disease (CJD) cases in the country and to study any possible link between CJD and BSE.

1992
Three in every 1,000 cows in the U.K. have BSE—the height of the epidemic.

1993
The 100,000th case of BSE in the U.K. is confirmed.

1995
Nineteen-year-old Stephen Churchill becomes the first victim of a new form of CJD: new variant Creutzfeldt-Jakob disease (nvCJD).

The Three Stages of Kuru

According to Dr. Gadjusek, there were three distinct stages of kuru. The first stage he called the ambulant stage (ambulant means that a patient is able to walk and is not confined to bed). During this stage, victims were unsteady on their feet, they started having trouble speaking, they shivered incessantly, and they lost coordination in their feet.

The second stage was called the sedentary stage (sedentary means spending a lot of the time sitting down). During this stage, victims became unable to walk, they lost control of their muscles, which would

1996
The export of British beef is banned by the European Union.

1997
British government researchers announce that there is "some evidence" that BSE can be passed from mother to calf.

1998
An official inquiry set up by the British government to investigate the spread of BSE and nvCJD begins collecting evidence.

1996
The total of nvCJD deaths reaches ten.

1996
British health minister Stephen Dorrell says that there is a "probable link" between BSE and nvCJD.

1997
A ban is introduced in the U.K. of the sale of all beef still on the bone.

also sometimes jerk uncontrollably, their moods and emotions would change drastically, and they would often burst out laughing for no reason. (This last symptom was why the disease was also known as the "laughing death" by the Foré.)

The third stage was called the terminal stage. In this stage, victims were unable to sit up without aid, their movements became even more uncontrollable, they had difficulty swallowing, and they developed ulcers. The patients would eventually die, but it would often take two years for this to happen. What made things more complicated was that the disease never appeared until at least two years after a person had

1999
The British government lifts the ban on the sale of beef on the bone.

2000
The first case of BSE in cows born in Germany.

2000
The first cases of BSE in Spain.

2000
The BSE inquiry publishes its report, which severely criticizes government ministers for their handling of the crisis.

2000
By December 2000, eighty-one people have died of nvCJD in the UK.

2001
Australia and New Zealand ban the import of beef from thirty European countries.

eaten a kuru-infected body part (and sometimes not until over twenty years later).

Against the Rules of Biology

We humans come equipped with a built-in defense mechanism of cells—called antibodies—whose job it is to attack diseases when they enter the bloodstream. Because of this, Dr. Gadjusek was dumbfounded by the fact that the antibodies weren't attacking and combating the virus. He reasoned that the virus might hide itself in, or with, something that the body thought was normal, and because it took so long to attack its victim, he called it a slow virus. However, the idea of a slow virus didn't seem to make complete sense. Eventually, researchers began to look for another way to explain what caused kuru and other TSEs.

Then, finally, in the early 1980s, an American scientist named Stanley B. Prusiner published an article in a scientific journal explaining that his team may have found the answer. However, if the idea of a slow virus didn't seem to make much sense, then to many scientists, Prusiner's answer seemed to make even less sense. What Prusiner had found went against all the rules of biology, and so it was that the idea of the prion came into being.

2

THE PROTEIN GOES BAD

Prior to Stanley B. Prusiner's article being published, everyone was wondering how a disease could exist without the body's defense system responding to it. But before we go on to describe Prusiner's discovery, we'll need to back up a bit.

How Diseases (Usually) Work

Diseases are normally caused by one of two things: either bacteria or viruses. Bacteria are single-celled organisms that exist everywhere—in the soil, in your body, in the air, in water. Often, they are very helpful to us (the bacteria in our intestines help us digest food), but some kinds of bacteria cause disease, such as salmonella, which is a severe form of food poisoning.

Viruses are microorganisms that are so small, they can't even be seen under normal microscopes. They need to live inside another organism—what scientists call the host—in order to survive. Viruses are generally made up of a strand of deoxyribonucleic acid (or DNA) that is covered by a layer of proteins, which helps to protect them. (We all have DNA—it's made up of genes, which help determine who we are and what we look like.) Viruses cause lots of diseases because they are parasitic, meaning that they usually hijack the cells of their host (maybe you) and then go on to damage the host's other cells, causing illness and sometimes death.

Prions: The Simple Protein Gone Wrong

A prion—"the answer" that scientist Stanley B. Prusiner came up with—is neither a virus nor a bacterium. In fact, it's much simpler than either: A prion is a protein. As was mentioned above, viruses are covered in protein; however, it's not just viruses that need proteins. Proteins are the building blocks of the body; muscles, for example, are 30 percent protein, and the liver is approximately 25 percent protein. Proteins also work as enzymes in our bodies, which means that they provoke chemical reactions. For example, french fries are full of complex carbohydrates and fats. When you eat fries, enzymes in your digestive system break down the complicated proteins in the carbohydrates into simple proteins that the body can use. Without enzymes, our bodies would stop being able to digest all the things needed in order to keep working. We can't make all the proteins we need, so we have to eat them; for example, soybeans and meat are full of proteins.

Each protein is made up of a long chain of amino acids. There are about twenty different common amino acids. They form various pro-

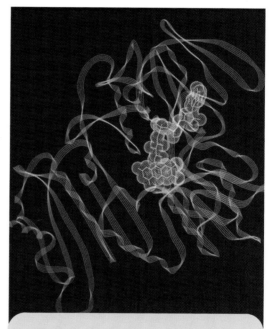

The helical structure of a protein, as seen under a microscope

teins, depending on which amino acids are linked together and in which order. If you looked at proteins under an incredibly powerful microscope, you would see that each protein is constructed in a spiral (what

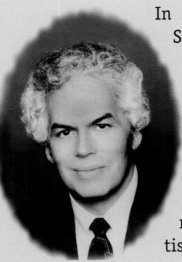

Dr. Stanley B. Prusiner

In 1972, an American doctor, Stanley B. Prusiner, treated a patient who eventually died from Creutzfeldt-Jakob disease. Dr. Prusiner was fascinated by TSEs and decided to investigate them. In 1974, he set up a laboratory and began his research. At the time, scientists were completely baffled as to what caused CJD. They thought that, like scrapie and kuru, CJD was caused by a "slow virus."

During his initial research, Dr. Prusiner read a report written in the 1960s by a team of scientists in London who were led by a doctor named Tikvah Alper. The team had taken tissue from scrapie-infected sheep and had exposed it to enough radiation to kill any known virus or bacterium. (Normally viruses die when they are exposed to radiation. This is because they contain a strand of DNA, and radiation destroys DNA.) But when Dr. Alper injected the tissue that had been exposed to radiation back into animals, the animals still died from scrapie. According to Dr. Alper, this meant that the infectious agent in scrapie did not contain any DNA. This was very, very strange because it was thought that all infectious agents had to have genetic material. Viruses take over cells by reproducing themselves, and to do so they need that little strand of DNA. How could an infectious agent reproduce if it didn't contain any DNA?

After experimenting on hamsters, Dr. Prusiner and his colleagues confirmed the findings of Dr. Alper—the normal methods used to kill viruses didn't affect the scrapie infectious agent. However, when they performed experiments that denatured proteins (a denatured protein can't do its job any longer), they found that the strength of the infectious agent was reduced. With this information in mind, they decided that what caused scrapie must mostly, if not totally, be made up of protein. Dr. Prusiner called the newly discovered infectious agent a prion. The name is a shortened version of its full name: proteinaceous infectious particle. (He rearranged the order a little; it should really be a proin.) Dr. Prusiner gave the prion protein the symbol PrP.

is called a helical structure). It would look like a corkscrew. And that's what a prion is. It's a simple protein—but it's a protein gone wrong.

Normal Versus Abnormal Prions

When Prusiner published his results in the journal *Science* in 1982, many scientists thought that he had gone mad. It seemed impossible that a protein could be an infectious agent. How did it spread? How did it reproduce itself? How come there were different versions of the protein in different TSEs? (Variation comes when things reproduce, and to do that DNA is needed.) But Prusiner kept on doing research, and soon he made another very important discovery. There are two types of prions: normal prions, which are good, and abnormal prions, which are bad. To differentiate between the two forms of the prions, he created two new symbols: PrPC for the normal prion and PrPSc for the abnormal prion (the Sc stands for scrapie, but it is now applied to all bad prions). The two prions seem to be exactly the same—they have exactly the same amino acids in exactly the same order—but in actuality, they have a different structure.

Like all proteins, a normal prion (PrPC) looks like a corkscrew; it has that same helical structure. A bad prion (PrPSc) has a flatter structure, and instead of looking like a corkscrew, it looks like a piece of string. To understand how a bad prion changes the structure of a normal prion, think of the prion proteins in your brain as a barrel of apples. Normally, a barrel of apples will remain edible for months, but if one rotten apple gets into the barrel, it will rot the apple next to it, which in turn will rot the apple next to it, and eventually, you end up with a barrel of bad apples. A PrPSc prion is like a bad apple, and bad prions spread not by replicating—or making copies of themselves—as a virus does, but by somehow converting the normal prion's helical structure into its own stringlike structure.

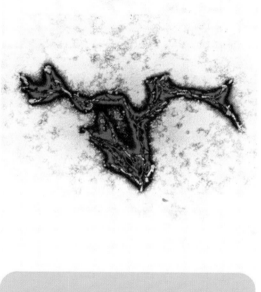

The PrPSc prion (pictured here) indicates Scrapie.

The helical structure of a normal protein makes it far less stable—it can be denatured easily by heat, acid, radiation, or enzymes. This is a good thing because it means that not only can a protein be easily broken down and used by the body but also that proteins do not build up where they shouldn't. In the brain, an enzyme called protease breaks down normal prions. Bad prions, however, can survive all of these things because their stringlike structure makes them much more stable; they just don't want to be denatured.

The different structures of the normal and abnormal prions may also explain why there are different strains of TSEs. Prusiner suggested that if a prion can have two different structures, why shouldn't it be able to have lots of different structures? It could have one specific structure in scrapie, for example, and another in BSE or CJD.

The Theory Behind How Prions Kill

There remains one big question: How do bad prions kill animals and humans?

The most accepted theory is that bad prions change the structure of normal prions in the neurons in the brain. Neurons are nerve cells that send electrical impulses from the brain to the rest of the body. When bad prions arrive in the brain, they can't be broken down by protease like normal prions. This means that they build up in the neurons to the point of causing blockage. Eventually, the neurons explode, leaving holes in the brain (the holes are like the craters left after a bomb has exploded), and with each explosion, the brain loses another messenger cell. The loss of the messenger cells becomes more serious as more parts of the body stop receiving messages about how to behave—and each time a neuron explodes, it releases its bad prions that go on to convert more normal prions. This theory also explains why it takes so long for TSEs to kill infected animals and people. Essentially, Prusiner's research indicates that it takes a long time for enough neurons to die to completely stop messages from going to the body's vital organs, such as the heart and lungs.

Now that the probable causes of the disease are established, let's return to cows. After all, they're the reason why so much research has been done on TSEs over the last twenty years.

3

THE COWS GO MAD

When Cow 133 died in 1985, scientists had no idea why. It was only in November 1986 that the disease we now know as BSE was officially recognized by British scientists. So how did this disease start and why did it spring up in the United Kingdom and not anywhere else?

More About Scrapie—the Oldest TSE

The oldest TSE is scrapie, which affects sheep and goats. It has been endemic (an endemic disease is one that is permanently in a population) in the United Kingdom for over 200 years. However, there is no proof that it has ever been passed to humans. One of the reasons for this has to do with the species barrier, meaning that it is difficult for diseases to spread from one species to another. Many people in the last 200 years have probably eaten sheep meat infected with scrapie, but because the disease was not strong enough to infect a human body, no one become ill.

However, experiments conducted with mice indicated that scrapie could infect other species aside from sheep. Scientists took the brains of sheep that had died from scrapie, mashed them up, and then injected them into the brains of mice. The mice got scrapie and died. (It has since been passed on to hamsters, rats, voles, gerbils, mink,

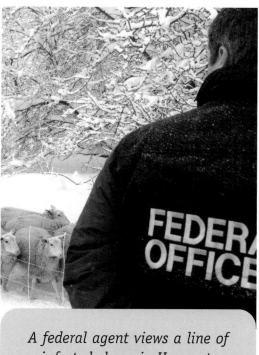

A federal agent views a line of infected sheep in Vermont.

and some species of monkey.) But there is a big difference between having infected brain injected into your own brain and eating infected meat. Sometime during the 1970s, scrapie appears to have become stronger, and according to many scientists, it managed to do what it had never done before: cross the species barrier and infect cows. It didn't do it alone, though. To cross that barrier, scrapie needed our help.

How Scrapie Crossed the Species Barrier

To understand the most commonly accepted theory about how scrapie crossed the species barrier, it's necessary to take a look at how a farm works and what farm animals eat.

The Farming Industry

Farmers need their livestock to grow quickly so that they can sell their meat and make a profit. A successful farmer needs cows that produce the maximum amount of milk. All of this is so that they can run their farming businesses efficiently and earn adequate money to keep the business profitable.

Since cows and sheep are herbivores, they eat plants and not meat. Animals (including farm animals) need protein in order to grow and be able to produce milk (just like us). However, most plants don't contain a lot of protein. Because of this, herbivores need to consume a huge amount of plants. To make things more efficient, farmers give their live-stock extra protein, and the cheapest and easiest way to do this is to recycle other animals (mostly cows and sheep, but other animals, too).

The Problem with Cannibalism . . .

Feeding extra protein to livestock meant that cows were eating sheep and other cows, and sheep were eating cows and other sheep. Farm animals had become carnivores and cannibals. This may seem hor-rible, but it actually makes sense. The protein that you can best digest (and the one that causes you to grow the quickest) is the one that comes from your own species. While in theory it should have been really good for cows to be eating cows, or sheep to be eating sheep, when you start to eat your own kind, like the Foré in Papua New Guinea did, problems can arise (which is why nature has taught most of us not to be cannibals).

When the MBM Went Bad

A disease gets weaker when it crosses the species bar-rier, but a disease gets stronger when it passes through the same species. For example, when kuru first became a problem among the Foré, the disease probably wasn't

When an animal is slaughtered, the meat is taken off the body. However, this still leaves the bits of animal that aren't normally consumed, such as the bones, the feet, and the head. These leftovers are rendered, meaning that everything is crushed and put in a giant vat, water is added, then it is all boiled. When the rendering process is over, a liquid sludge remains made up of protein with a layer of fat floating on the top. When the two are separated (the fat is used in a variety of products, such as washing powder), the protein sludge is dried out and turned into what is known as meat-and-bone meal, or MBM.

When fed to animals, MBM is an easy and inexpensive way to provide the livestock with lots of extra protein. About 10 million tons of animal protein is produced each year in the world, most of it in North America, western Europe, and Australia, and about 5.5 million tons of that (or just over half) is fed to animals as feed.

MBM protein was first widely used in the United Kingdom during World War II. During the war, it was very difficult for

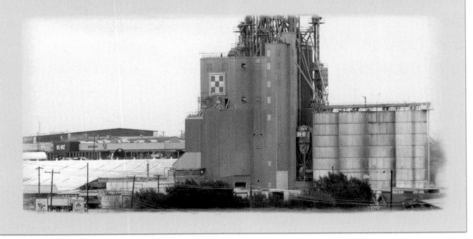

Britain to get enough vegetable protein for the country's livestock, so farmers started feeding them MBM, which was cheap and plentiful. This practice continued for decades in Britain. MBM was also given to cows in the United States, but far less frequently than in Britain. Eventually, the cost of rendering become too high—it takes a lot of fuel to keep a giant vat of animal waste boiling—and a cheaper method was needed. During the 1970s, the rendering industry came up with a system that used a vacuum—a space where there is no air. When water is heated in a vacuum, it boils at a lower temperature, hence using less energy. This seemed like a great solution. But there was a problem, which wouldn't be immediately obvious.

very strong. However, as more people ate more people who had died from the disease, the disease became stronger and more concentrated—and the stronger the disease, the easier it is for it to jump from one species to another.

Back in the time when the remains of sheep were still boiled at high temperatures in the United Kingdom, the scrapie prion was killed (not even a bad prion can survive the heat of a rendering vat). Scientists believe that when the temperatures were lowered, the stable scrapie prion wasn't killed and it remained in the MBM. Hence, the animals who were being fed MBM were also eating scrapie prions. The more the sheep ate scrapie-infested MBM, the stronger it got. And as it got stronger, it became more likely that scrapie would make the jump from sheep and goats to another animal. When the scrapie prion did make the jump, it jumped to the animals who were eating the most MBM—cows—and it was at this point that scrapie became bovine spongiform encephalopathy, or BSE. The trouble was that at the time, no one realized this was happening.

The Birth of Bovine Spongiform Encephalopathy

In the United Kingdom, the jump was probably made in the early 1980s, but since at that point no one knew about the disease, the infected cattle were probably sent to be rendered into MBM. This MBM was then fed to more cows that died and were then rendered into MBM—and so the cycle continued. With most of the cows in the country being fed MBM, you can see how the disease could spread.

In November 1986, when BSE was finally recognized as a disease and was given its name, scientists didn't know where it had come from. Because of this, in May 1987, the government's center for animal diseases—the Central Veterinary Laboratory—was asked to investigate. It spent six months looking into the situation before discovering that the disease was being spread by infected MBM.

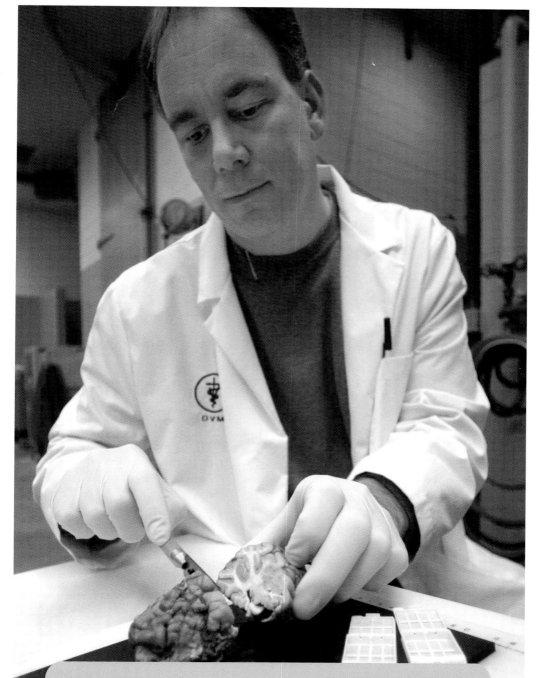

Veterinarian Dr. Dave Steffen extracts brain tissue to test it for bovine spongiform encephalopathy.

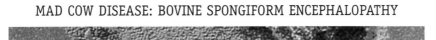

The Spread of BSE

Meanwhile, the number of cows being diagnosed with the disease in the United Kingdom kept on growing. Before 1988, there were 446 confirmed cases of the disease. In 1988, there were 2,514; in 1989, there were 7,228; in 1990, there were 14,407; in 1991, there were 25,359; in 1992, there were 37,280. The British government introduced a series of measures to try to stop the spread of the disease. They banned the use of MBM for cows and sheep; they said that any cattle found to have the disease should immediately be slaughtered and then burned; they made BSE a "notifiable disease," which meant that any case had to be reported immediately to the government's vets; they stopped milk from infected cows from being fed to other cows. However, the disease kept appearing, and by 1993, over 100,000 cases of BSE had been confirmed.

Humans at Risk?

It is not totally unheard of for diseases to cross from animals to humans (these kinds of diseases are called zoonotic diseases). Influenza is thought to have crossed over from pigs to humans, and it's thought that smallpox crossed over to humans from cows. Despite this, scientists did not think that BSE posed a threat to human health when it first broke out in cattle. Scientists, who were aware that scrapie had never affected humans, decided that BSE was probably the same. They believed that it would stay in cows and would not cross the species barrier—that there was nothing to worry about.

Then, in 1990, five antelopes living in British zoos died, and it was discovered that their brains resembled those of cows that had died from BSE. Later that year (also in Britain), a domestic cat fell ill and died. It, too, had a brain that looked like it had been infected with BSE.

It suddenly seemed that the risk to human health might be much greater than had been previously thought. BSE seemed to cross the species barrier easily. That left just one question: How long would it take before the disease made the jump to humans?

4

THE FINAL FRONTIER

Beef is big business. British beef was exported all over the world, from Austria to Australia, from the Azores to the Falklands; it supported thousands of jobs in the country. Since this was the case, the British government was desperate to reassure the public that beef was safe to eat. In 1990, the minister of agriculture, John Gummer, invited newspapers and TV stations to a press conference and fed a hamburger to his four-year-old daughter, Cordelia, in front of the journalists. At the same time that the government was telling the public that things were fine, they had also set up a research unit at the University of Edinburgh in Scotland. The CJD Surveillance Unit was set up to examine every case of CJD and see if there were any new variations—variations that might indicate that BSE had made the species barrier jump. Despite what the government was saying and despite the measures it had taken to combat the disease, eating beef definitely wasn't safe.

Specified Bovine Offal

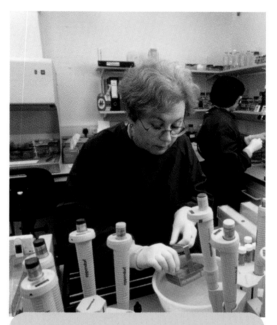

In cows, BSE takes about five years to appear. However, because at the time there was no way to test animals for BSE infection, the only way to know that a cow was infected was when it showed symptoms. The government banned the sale to the public of what they called "specified bovine offal," which included the head, the spinal cord, and the eyes—all the bits of the cow that were thought to hold the most danger of infecting people.

A technician checks brain tissue for new variant Creutzfeldt-Jakob disease, the human disease linked to mad cow.

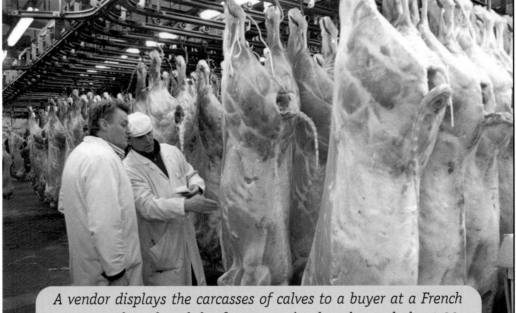

A vendor displays the carcasses of calves to a buyer at a French meat market, though beef consumption has dropped about 30 percent since British beef was banned from continental Europe.

It is now thought that over 700,000 BSE-infected cows were slaughtered and then eaten by humans between 1990 and 1996. It takes only a quarter of a gram of BSE-infected cow to infect another cow (a piece about the size of a peppercorn), and while it takes more than that to infect a human (how much more is not known), it wasn't long before BSE did what scrapie had never managed to do: BSE began killing people.

To Eat Beef, or Not to Eat Beef . . . That Is the Question

On March 20, 1996, the minister of health for the British government, Stephen Dorrell, stood up in the House of Commons, one of the branches of the British

In 1994, eighteen-year-old Stephen Churchill became ill. He started hallucinating (seeing things that weren't there), and he stopped talking to his family. He began to tremble and make jerky movements. Before long, he was taken to the hospital where he began to lose weight. Finally, he fell into a coma, and on May 21, 1995, he died.

Because it is so unusual for CJD to strike anyone who is so young, the CJD Surveillance Unit was alerted. Scientists found a blob of protein on Stephen's brain that didn't look like those found on the brains of people who had died from normal CJD. The protein was in a different part of the brain as well. In normal CJD, most of the damage to the brain is in the cerebrum, which is the front part of the brain, but with the new disease, the damage was concentrated in the cerebellum, which is at the back of the brain. The blobs of protein—or protein plaques, as scientists call them—were also larger and more rounded than normal, and the telltale holes (or vacuoles) were lined up around the plaques. Scientists thought that this arrangement looked like a daisy, and because of this, they called each plaque a florid plaque. (Florid comes from the Latin word for flower.) All of this resulted in the brain looking like the brain of a cow that had died from BSE.

The disease that had killed Stephen Churchill was named new variant Creutzfeldt-Jakob disease, or nvCJD. (It is always written with a lowercase *nv* and uppercase *CJD*.) Armed with their new evidence, the scientists told the government that they had better warn the public.

Parliament. Dorrell told the members gathered that although there was no proof that there was a link between BSE and nvCJD, "the most likely explanation at present is that these cases are linked to exposure to BSE." The government had finally told the public that eating beef might well be dangerous.

The proof of a link came soon afterward, when chemical analysis showed that brain samples from the brains of nvCJD victims had exactly the same molecular structure as the brains of cows that had died from BSE.

Why the Infected Beef Didn't Kill Everyone

Simply proving that the diseases were one and the same did not help show how people had become infected in the first place. There are hundreds of thousands, possibly millions, of British people who ate infected beef during the 1980s, but not all of them have contracted nvCJD. Why? One of the reasons is that it is probably quite difficult for the prion to get to the brain. In experiments conducted in order to see if TSEs can be passed from one species to another, researchers most often inject infected material into the brains of other animals. This is, in a way, cheating—injecting material directly into the place where it is going to do the most

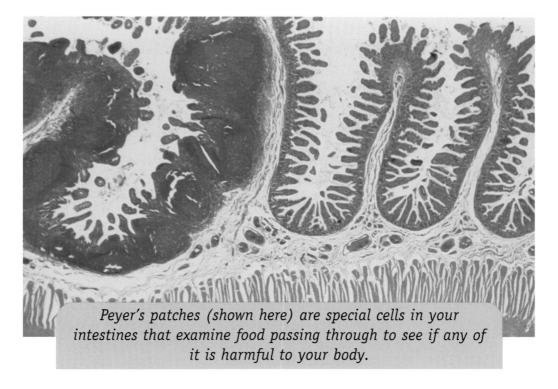

Peyer's patches (shown here) are special cells in your intestines that examine food passing through to see if any of it is harmful to your body.

harm. In humans, though, the prions contained in the infected material are eaten. This means that somehow the prions have to get from the intestines—your stomach and guts—to your brain. How that happens is— yes, you've guessed it—a mystery.

Peyer's Patch

The most accepted theory goes like this. You eat some infected meat, which passes from your stomach into your gut. The enzymes that normally break down proteins in your gut don't work on the bad prion. Meanwhile, on the walls of your intestines are little knots of tissue (or nodules) called Peyer's patches. These are part of your body's immune, or defense, system. On the surface of the Peyer's patches are special cells that capture bits of broken-down food in your intestines and examine them to see if they might contain anything that could harm the body. Scientists think that the bad prions get into the bodies of cows and sheep through the Peyer's patches, and that it's likely to be the same for humans. A bad prion can pass by this line of the body's defenses because it's a protein (even if it's a bad one) and so it's not noticed. Scientists believe that the prions then move to the spleen (another part of the body's immune system that breaks down blood cells). They then move through the nerves and up the spine before finally arriving at the brain. (That might explain why the damage is caused at the back of the brain— the prions arrive and stay in the first bit of brain they find.) Once in your brain, there's only one thing that's going to happen: You're going to die.

Another Theory: Codon 129

There is, however, another possible reason that explains why BSE has not infected more people with nvCJD. A PrPC prion is made up of 253 amino acids (remember that all proteins are made from long chains of amino acids). At position (or codon as it's properly known) 129 of that long chain, there can be two amino acids—either methionine or valine, or both.

You have two copies of the gene (genes are what make up DNA) that creates PrPC, one from your mother and one from your father. At codon 129 of the chain, you might have inherited either two methionine amino acids, two valines, or one of each. Everybody who has died from nvCJD has had two methionine amino acids at codon 129 and this has led scientists to speculate that a person's chances of contracting nvCJD depend on the makeup of his or her codon 129.

Scientists think that if you have one methionine and one valine at codon 129, then you're largely protected from the disease; if you have two valines, you are more vulnerable; if you have two methionines, then you are most likely to be infected.

In the United Kingdom, it is believed that 40 percent of the population has two methionine amino acids at codon 129. That means that 24 million people are vulnerable.

Mad Cow on the Move

Since the disease killed Stephen Churchill in 1995, nvCJD has killed over ninety more people and the number keeps on rising. Most of these deaths have been in the United Kingdom, but there have also been deaths in France and Ireland. (To find out the number of deaths in the United Kingdom, you can visit

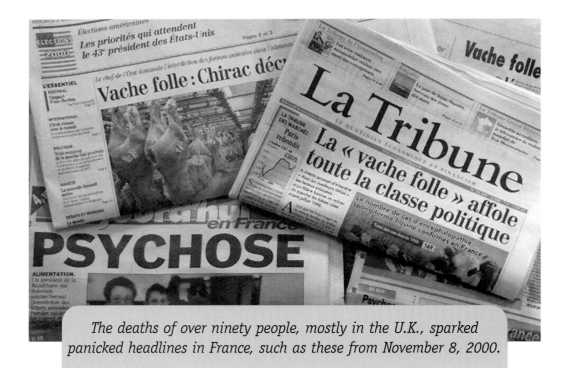

The deaths of over ninety people, mostly in the U.K., sparked panicked headlines in France, such as these from November 8, 2000.

the U.K. Department of Health's Web site, which is listed in the For More Information section in the back of this book.) What is not known is how many people the disease is eventually going to kill.

Estimates change all the time because no one knows how long the infection stays in the body before beginning to have an effect. At one point, scientists who worked for the European Community said that one infected cow could infect 500,000 people. This is now thought to be an overestimate. The latest research suggests that the eventual figure will be 136,000 deaths in the United Kingdom from the disease. Perhaps the only slightly reassuring thing is that we're not cannibals. The disease infected so many cows because they were eating other BSE-infected cows, which allowed the disease to get stronger and infect over 160,000 cows. Because we're not eating victims of nvCJD, our chances are probably better. But that's not much comfort for those people who may have eaten beef infected with BSE.

If you live in the United States, chances are you have never eaten infected beef, but that doesn't mean that you shouldn't be careful, as we'll see in the next chapter.

5

ARE WE SAFE?

Since BSE was discovered in the United Kingdom, it has spread to Germany, France, Portugal, Spain, Switzerland, the Netherlands, Belgium, Denmark, Luxembourg, Oman, the Falkland Islands, and the Azores. There has also been one case in Canada. Experts think that it will appear in other countries because infected MBM was exported to over eighty countries around the world. (Over 600,000 tons went to Indonesia alone.)

Mad Cow in the United States: The Government Reacts

The U.S. government was quick to react to the threat posed by BSE. So far, there has been no sign of BSE in American cattle, but that's not to say that it couldn't happen.

- In 1989, the government stopped "live ruminants" from being imported from countries that had cases of BSE. (Ruminants are animals such as cows, sheep, antelopes, deer, or giraffes.)

- Also banned was the importation of products made from ruminants, such as fats or MBM.

- Anyone who had spent more than six months in the United Kingdom between 1980 and 1996 was banned from donating blood. (It's still not certain that the disease can be spread through blood, but it's better to be safe.)

- Once it was discovered that MBM was the origin of BSE in the United Kingdom, sheep or cow-based MBM was not allowed to be fed to sheep or cows.

MBM With and Without Sheep and Cows

The U.S. government, however, has permitted farmers to keep using this kind of MBM for pigs and chickens. (They don't appear to get BSE.) In regard to the factories that produce MBM, past experience in the U.K. has shown that it is very difficult to stop the two products—MBM that doesn't contain any sheep or cows and MBM that does—from being mixed together. This is called cross contamination, and in the United Kingdom, from 1988 to 1996, it is estimated that over 60,000 cows were infected by cross-contaminated MBM.

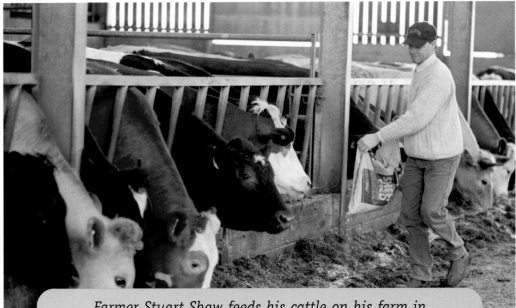

Farmer Stuart Shaw feeds his cattle on his farm in Staffordshire, England, in the wake of a BSE outbreak.

And it's not just the factories. If you're a farmer and you receive two loads of MBM, one for your cows and one for your pigs, you probably store all your feed in the same place. What's to stop the two getting mixed up or one kind being fed to the wrong animal? And since it has been shown that TSE prions can be eaten by an animal without making it sick (like scrapie prions in humans), why couldn't a pig become infected with BSE and then get turned into feed for cows?

Downer Cattle Only

Another worry is that, according to some specialists, the main reason that no case of BSE has ever been found in the United States is simply because the government isn't looking hard enough. In the United States, the only cattle tested for BSE are what are known as downer cattle—cattle that can no longer walk or are sick. By the end of 2000, 11,953 brains from downer cattle had been examined for BSE by the government and no sign of BSE was found. That is fine, except that, as we've mentioned before, there's no way to know if a cow is infected by BSE until it starts showing symptoms—unless it's tested. (A test for BSE has been developed since the first outbreak in the U.K.)

BSE Tests in the European Union

Though unlikely, it is possible that, just as in the U.K., infected cattle could end up being eaten by humans. The European Union was so worried that this might continue to happen there, it decided that as of June 2001, all cattle over thirty months of age would have to be tested for BSE. Some countries, such as France and Germany, introduced testing before the deadline and in the first three months of testing, the German government found nine cases of BSE. During 2000, when the policy was simply testing downer cattle—as it is here—they found only seven cases during the entire year.

BSE in American Cattle—It May Be Hard to Recognize

Though the U.S. government has banned all imports of cow products from the countries where BSE has been reported, there's another way that BSE could spring up. As we saw earlier, 85 percent of CJD cases break out randomly—about 250 human cases a year in the United States. Scientists think that rates of random animal TSEs occur with about the same frequency. For this reason, it's possible that the disease is already striking approximately 100 cattle a year. If these cows are made into MBM, which is then eaten by other cows, it could provoke the same situation that occurred in the United Kingdom.

Also, it is possible that scientists are simply not recognizing BSE in American cattle because it might be found here in a different form. In 1979, scientists injected the brains of sheep that had died from scrapie in the United States into the brains of cattle. Not all of the cows developed the disease, but three did. The disease they developed was bovine spongiform encephalopathy, but it was different from the disease that was seen in Europe. American cows infected with American scrapie developed a specific American BSE. So if the government is looking for BSE that resembles the British or European version, then they might well miss cases.

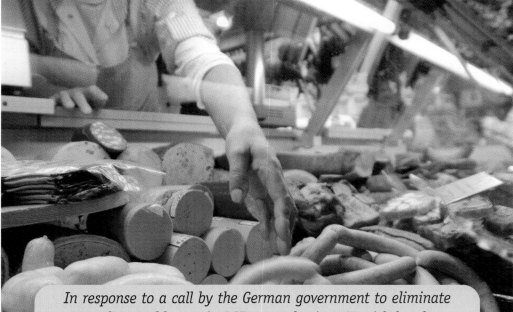

In response to a call by the German government to eliminate meat that could contain BSE, a vendor in a Munich butchery restocks the cooling shelf with new sausage.

The Meat You Eat

If BSE does exist without anyone knowing about it, the meat you eat could be dangerous. Meats such as steak are mainly muscle, and scientists think that it is almost impossible to be infected with BSE from muscle. (Prions don't gather there.) However, when these cuts of meat have been taken from the body of a cow, there are bits left over. One place where leftover meat is found is around the spinal cord. It's difficult to cut this meat off, so in the United States, this kind of meat is forced off the spinal cord at high pressure. The meat collected is called mechanically separated meat, and it's used in lots of products, such as canned spaghetti sauce or hot dogs (which can contain up to 20 percent mechanically separated meat).

According to the World Health Organization, which is part of the United Nations, the brain, the spinal cord, and the eyes are the most dangerous parts of a cow infected with BSE. The lungs, the liver, the kidneys, the spleen, the fluid that surrounds the spinal cord, and the placenta—the sac that surrounds a calf in its mother's body—are also dangerous, but less so.) If any BSE prions are lurking in a cow, then the spinal cord is one of the places where you're most likely to find them. Any meat taken from the spinal cord is likely to be infected.

All of this might leave you asking one question: Am I in danger? Sadly, there's only one answer: It's impossible to really know. As you've seen in this book, there are no clear answers with bovine spongiform encephalopathy or with new variant Creutzfeldt-Jakob disease. Scientists are working hard to gain a better understanding of this horrible disease, but research takes time, especially when you are investigating a disease that can take many years to show itself. There has been much progress in the last twenty-five years, but there are still no definite answers. We'll all have to wait and see.

GLOSSARY

amino acids Basic components of proteins.

bovine spongiform encephalopathy (BSE) TSE that infects cows.

Britain Nation of Great Britain, made up of England, Scotland, and Wales.

chronic wasting disease (CWD) TSE that infects deer and elk.

Creutzfeldt-Jakob disease (CJD) Human TSE that infects about 250 people a year in the United States.

kuru TSE that affected the Foré people of Papua New Guinea. It was spread by the practice of cannibalism. The word means "to shiver" or "to tremble" in the Foré's language.

meat-and-bone meal (MBM) Livestock feed that is manufactured from the remains of slaughtered livestock but that cannot be directly consumed by humans. It is fed to livestock as a source of protein.

nvCJD New variant Creutzfeldt-Jakob disease, the TSE caused by eating beef infected with BSE.

prion Naturally occurring protein that, when structurally altered, is believed to be the disease-causing agent of all TSEs. The name was coined by American scientist Stanley B. Prusiner and is short for proteinaceous infectious particle.

protein Set of amino acids; vital part of all living organisms.

PrPC Normal prion protein with a helical structure.

PrPSc Disease-causing prion protein with a string-like structure.

transmissible mink encephalopathy (TME) TSE that infects mink.

transmissible spongiform encephalopathies (TSEs) Group of diseases that cause the appearance of protein plaques and holes in the brain of their victims. All TSEs are fatal.

FOR MORE INFORMATION

Centers for Disease Control
Web site: http://www.cdc.gov/ncidod/diseases/cjd/
    bse_cjd_qa.htm
Frequently asked questions about BSE and CJD.

The European Commission
Web site: http://www.europa.eu.int/comm/food/fs/
    bse/index_en.html

Food and Drug Administration
Web site: http://www.fda.gov
Recent information on mad cow disease can be
found on the FDA home page.

United Kingdom Department of Health
Web site: http://www.doh.gov.uk/cjd/cjd_stat.htm
For the latest figures on nvCJD victims in the
United Kingdom.

United States Department of Agriculture (USDA)
Web site: http://www.usda.gov.
Recent updates on food safety and BSE.

University of Illinois at Urbana-Champaign
BSE Information at UIUC
Web site: http://w3.aces.uiuc.edu/AnSci/BSE

World Health Organization's fact sheet on BSE
Web site: http://www.who.int/inf-fs/en/fact113.html
World Health Organization's fact sheet
    on nvCJD.
Web site: http://www.who.int/inf-fs/en/fact180.html

World Organization of Animal Health
Web site: http://www.oie.int/eng/info/
    en_esbmonde.htm
For the latest figures on BSE cases around the world.

FOR FURTHER READING

Klitzman, Robert. *The Trembling Mountain: A Personal Account of Kuru, Cannibals, and Mad Cow Disease.* New York: Plenum Trade, 1998.

Rampton, Sheldon, and John Stauber, eds. *Mad Cow U.S.A.* Monroe, ME: Common Courage Press, 1997.

Ratzan, Scott C., ed. *Mad Cow Crisis: Health and the Public Good.* New York: New York University Press, 1998.

Rhodes, Richard. *Deadly Feasts: The "Prion" Controversy and the Public's Health.* New York: Touchstone Books, 1998.

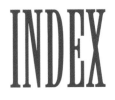

INDEX

CREDITS

About the Author

Tom Ridgway lives and works in Paris, France, and has probably eaten BSE-infected beef.

Photo Credits

Cover and chapter title interior photos © Em Unit, VLA/Science Photo Library; pp. 4, 6, 12, 15, 34, 42, 52, 55 © AP/Wide World Photo; p. 10 © Dean Conger/Corbis; pp. 13, 27 © Custom Medical Stock Photo; p. 23 © Will & Deni McIntyre; p. 24 © Corbis; pp. 31, 48 © Agence France Presse/Corbis; p. 37 © AP/Lincoln Journal Star; p. 41 © James King/Holmes Science Library; p. 45 © Biophoto Associates.

Series Design

Evelyn Horovicz

Layout

Les Kanturek